My Amazing True Experience with Keto diet and intermittent fasting

My weight loss story: how I lost 40 pounds in 3 months by combining Keto diet and intermittent fasting

My personal case study as I followed a diet plan that made me lose 40 pounds in 3 months without any exercise, just changing what I eat and when I eat. How I lost my cravings and hunger, and how this healthy lifestyle is more satisfying and fulfilling than eating normal food. How this diet is the best way to improve your immune system and overall health to combat diseases, cancer and outbreaks like the Current global outbreak.

I will tell you my story before the diet, how I found the information, how I applied the information, benefits of keto, benefits of intermittent fasting, my plan, and my results. Things I didn't do during my diet that I can recommend you do which will help you greatly in achieving better results. Also I have a word of advice to you as your fellow human been.

My story before the diet

I started the diet at the beginning of December 2019. I'm 5.7 feet (175 centimeters) and before the diet I was 205 pounds (93 kilo grams). I never stopped eating. There was always something in my mouth, as I just quitted smoking and I needed to keep my mouth occupied, and food is the best thing to make your mouth busy. I had a huge belly, someone told me I was pregnant in a triplet. I had some fats in my arms, legs, face, thighs, and love handles. Everyone told me your body shape is ugly, as my mid-section was not in harmony with the rest of my body. My wife pushed me so hard to do exercises to lose weight and be fit and lean. I have been an accountant for more than a decade, that job made me sit all the time, eat a lot and rarely do any activities.

I ate all kind of junk food, fast food, desserts, canned and processed food, always drinking sodas and canned juices, I ate so much manufactured food and snacks. I ate 4 or 5 meals a day plus 2 to 3 snacks. I used to go to the supermarket every night and got potato chips, biscuits, juices, sodas, snacks. I loved eating and was a big foody. It gave me pleasure and satisfaction. Frustration, depression, sadness, and many other negative mental feelings related to life disappointed made me ate more.

Eating was an addiction for me. It was a mental and psychological dysfunction. My body was always forcing me to operate my mouth and fill my stomach no matter what the consequences were, whether I was hungry or not. Just for the sake of feeling full and satisfied. If I saw food, I immediately put it in my mouth and without hesitation I swallow it.

I always had headaches, high blood pressure. My last blood test showed that I had gout and high Cholesterol. I made X-ray scan and found out that I had a fatty liver. I made stool test and found that I had dangerously low digestive functions. My body was screaming for help and most of my organs were not functioning properly. I was always lazy and found it hard to move or do activities. Fatigue was my companion all day, every day.

I had brain fog, and my memory was weak. I had acidity in my stomach, I felt it in constant basis. There was inflammation in my guts most of the time, bloating after eating and all kinds of digestive problems. My Intestines painfully had gas most of the time. My breathing was not normal, and my sight was getting weaker. I had so many problems and I went to few different doctors. They gave me medicine and advised me to change my diet. The medicine did not work, and I did not go through with their diet advice.

It was very hard for me to change my eating habits. I was in denial of my eating disorder and my body was paying the price. My life as a whole suffered. My work life and my performance and productivity were declining. I often had arguments about my health and bed performance with my wife. Everyone was urging me to act and just to start to change this aspect of my life.

After so long I finally decided to do something about. I thought about where to start. Most people told me you need to work out, maybe I should do some weightlifting, cardio, aerobics or high intensity interval training. I tried some of those, but nothing seemed to work. I was always tired and exhausted and couldn't finish any exercise. And after every workout I was so hungry that I ate more.

This approach to the problem was completely wrong and I gave up quickly. I thought working out is the key to weight loss and to have a healthier life; and failing to do so left broken and depressed even more. I lacked confidence and I was destroyed emotionally.

After some time I decided to go back on the hunt for information that would eventually get me to lose weight.

How I found the information

Of course on the internet. I'm and addict to YouTube; I can watch it for hours tirelessly. I accidently came across the phrases "intermittent fasting" and "ketogenic diet". I started digging and found many youtubers talking about the infinite benefits of those two plans.

I started following some of those self-proclaimed expert youtubers and I found out that they have so much information on the subject matter. They had a great way of preaching their ways based on science and proven official researches. They had years of experience, trial and error. Their CVs were rich in previous cases they helped to achieve what they were promising.

Those youtubers are, in no specific order:

1- Dr. Eric Berg: probably my favorite. I learned a lot from him. He is the best. He has this way of speaking and making the information go straight to your heart and get it imprinted on your memory. He has decades of experience on the above mentioned two phrases. His motto is "don't lose weight to be healthy, but it the other way around, eat healthy then you will lose weight"; or it is something similar, I can't remember the exact quote.

2- Thomas Delauer: this guy is the real deal. He is a celebrity health trainer and renowned coach. He is the fact guy, as he always gets his information and facts from medical researches published by well-reputed organizations and universities. He keeps you updated on all trends and recent researches and other published medical information related to the subject matter. He is the personification of a successful weight loss experience.

3- Gravity Transformation - Fat Loss Experts: this is a great channel to get all sorts of information regarding everything related to weight loss, not just the above mentioned two "phrases". They have plenty of plans and diet systems you can benefit from to lose weight. They talk a lot about keto and fasting but also other things as well that will help you get the best healthy lifestyle.

4- Dr. Nick Zyrowski: he has a great channel in which he talks about the subject matter and all things related to healthy eating. He has big experience in nutrition and diets, as well as utilizing the science of food for a better life overall.

5- Dr Sam Robbins" another channel with great information on all health-related issues. He has a great database of videos that will help you greatly in losing weight and living a healthy life. His main focus is to get stronger, healthier, fitter and leaner. Also he is in the game of nutrition and healthy food based on scientific facts and findings. He is strong in the medical field and knows a lot about the industry of medicine.

6- Dr. Sten Ekberg: his channel is similar in some ways to Dr. Eric Berg's in how he presents his knowledge and the information presented. He has a deep understanding of how the body works, and how it reacts to food consumption. This is a great channel for weight loss and living the healthy lifestyle, with huge information about keto and fasting.

The best thing about all of those channels that they have thousands of hours of free content that you need not to pay a dime to get. They promote, recommend and vouch for other paid courses and health products that I advise you give it a try based on your needs and requirements.

I'm not promoting them or their products, but I recommend that you follow them, and you will learn a lot from them. You can subscribe to their channels, follow them on Twitter and Instagram and like their Facebook pages. They are great personalities and have a presence online as health gurus and influencers, and the information you gather from them will help you a lot in your quest for a healthy lifestyle. Either you use and follow my specific method of weight loss, or you learn many methods and approaches from them and gather as much information as you can, and then construct your own diet and plan.

What made that method the best approach for me to learn and apply for my weight loss quest was that I considered those youtubers as my mentors. My schedule and my wallet couldn't afford a real-time coach or trainer. I loved watching them, it was a pleasure hearing them and learning from them. They were like my dad or bro. I took their words seriously and felt they did care about me. They made me appreciate my body and be confident again about it. They opened my eyes on my potentials and on all the wonders inside the miraculous machine that is the human body. They took my hand and guided me to find the path to my goal.

I used to watch YouTube for the funny clips, vlogs, celebrity gossips, news, trailers, debates, and other types of videos. Now my main interest in YouTube is to watch the new content the above mentioned youtubers are putting out and to learn from it. That subject is now of the most interest and excitement to me, and it helps me a lot.

There are many other channels in YouTube with so much information. You can subscribe to them all, but it is better to follow as few as possible to not get lost in that ocean of information. Also there are so many different and contradicting opinions, so you need to trust the right people so you would not end up with the wrong information and misleading facts.

How I applied the information

I watched hundreds of videos about Keto and fasting, and other general health issues related to weight loss. I wrote down in a word document on my laptop all the important information that might help, things like:

- The best healthy food that will have the strongest effect on my overall health. There are super foods that everyone needs to consume to have the largest amount of nutrition. There are certain foods that have so many minerals, vitamins and other substances that the body needs to function properly at maximum capacity. Foods like avocado, broccoli, garlic and Kale are great in preventing diseases and are loaded with minerals and vitamins.
- When to eat. This is as important as what to eat. I don't want to get technical as I'm not an expert. However, the timing of eating has a significant impact on your overall health and your weight loss aspirations. There are many approaches to this dilemma, and it differs from person to persons, and it is based on the diet you will apply.
- The benefits about each food and pattern. I needed to determine the benefits of each factor I would include in the diet. Ketogenic diet has many variances and ways to approach and implement it. I needed to figure out the best technique attainable and applicable for me. The same goes for intermittent fasting.

- Habits and rituals and how to change them. Those videos mainly talk about foods, nutrition, and other health subjects, but sometimes they talk about the mental health as well. You need to be physically and mentally prepared for what to come. It is a battle of wills and you need to be ready for it. You will be hungry, and there is a slight chance you might get sick for different reasons if you start changing your eating habits and food rituals. But the end result is most rewarding, and your goal is worth fighting for. Those videos encourage you, push you forward, support you, enlighten you, and give you the hope of a better tomorrow. You just need to step up and seize the opportunity.

I compiled a list of all the information I needed and started applying what I knew, and I came up with a plan. I estimated my potentials and how I would go through and survive such a strict eating plan. I know myself and know what would lift me up and what would break me down. I needed to do this and go through with it till the end.

You need to do the same. You need to know what foods are best for you. Maybe you are allergic to something I'm consuming. Maybe you don't like to eat something I love to eat.

You should measure your weight and height, how much calories you need to consume daily to start to lose weight. You can scientifically approach this matter or just leave it to be and stop your unhealthy food habits and start eating healthy and do fasting. Either ways are working, and you will see results.

My plan

It is very simple and straight forward. You can follow it entirely or you can pick and choose what fits your budget and schedule and benefits you the most.

Every weekly off day I go to the grocery and buy vegetables, fruits, beef, chicken, fish, and other food items. I go home and I prepare a 7 days meal plan. My diet was almost the same on weekly basis, but I tweaked it occasionally.

For the seven days ahead, I prepared salad and seasoned my beef and chicken. I made all food items and supplements ready for consumption. I had an air fryer, which helped me a lot in eating healthy food. All fried chicken, potatoes and other fried foods where cooked in the air fryer with just adding one tablespoon of olive oil or unsalted butter.

For my off and on hours, I usually slept for 7 to 8 hours continuously and never got naps. Sleeping enough period of time is most beneficial for dozens of reasons. It helps on so many health issues, especially of course weight loss, combined with other techniques.

For the first couple of months I slept at 11:30 pm and woke up at 7:30 am. Then I kept moving my sleeping timing earlier till I reached 9:30 pm and waked up 5:00 am. The less I ate the better my sleep was. My plan dictated that the last thing I ate was before at least 90 minutes before my bedtime, otherwise I got trouble sleeping or waking up on tome.

I don't eat anything until 1 pm. This is an intermittent fasting pattern I applied for that period of time. This was when I did 8 hours of eating window and followed it by 16 hours of fasting window. On those 8 hours I ate 3 meals and on the 16 hours I didn't eat anything at all.

In the 16 hours fasting window I only drank two small or medium cups coffee and green tea on daily basis, without sugar or milk or cream. I sometimes consumed a third cup of herbal tea, black tea, ginger, cinnamon or mint, boiled in a cup of water, and also without any sugar. I sometimes added Stevia sweetener.

It was hard at first to skip breakfast till launch time. I didn't give up on my breakfast entirely, I just delayed it few hours. From 1 pm till 9 pm I ate the 3 meals. I needed to prolong the fasting period.

Since I woke up till 1 pm I don't eat anything, I just drank coffee and tea, all black without any sugar, sweeteners, milk or cream. Again this is very important, otherwise you will ruin the fasting.

On 1 pm I ate breakfast, which is 3 half boiled eggs. Eggs has so much nutrition benefits and made me feel full for a long period of time.

On 4 pm I ate salad and protein. The protein was diverse every day. Sometimes I ate chicken breasts, other times I ate grilled beef or steak. Few times I ate grilled fish, like salmon, sardine or just any filleted fish. It is advices to consume fats with protein in a high-fat diet, and the best type of fat to include in your diet is the organic and natural fats that come with the beef and chicken.

The salad consisted of 10 items which are, cucumber, cherry tomato, green pepper, carrot, lettuce, kale, avocado, broccoli, parsley, Rocca or rocket leaves. You need to include as much green leaves in your salad as humanly possible, especially cruciferous veggies. The salad plate ingredients eventually weighted half a pound.

I put on the salad half tablespoon that included sea salt, black pepper, red pepper, one tablespoon of olive oil and apple cider vinegar, and one lemon.

My dinner was some nuts and fruits and I started eating it at 8 pm. I consumed nuts like almond, hazelnut, pistachio, walnuts and cashew. The fruits I consumed varied hugely, but my main go to were orange, apple, banana, and all kinds of berries. Sometimes I drank milk or ate yogurt, low fat and pasteurized.

I sometimes made pasta with cream sauce or tomato sauce. I sometimes consumed popcorn.

And by sometimes, I mean once or twice weekly.

Those were what I ate during the evening. On that 8 hours window I consumed food only and drank some water. The water was never an issue for me, and I didn't consume certain amount of it. Whenever I felt hungry or thirsty, I drank water.

I stopped eating at 9 pm and went to sleep at 11:30 pm. During those 2 and half hours I drank water, green tea and one tablespoon of apple cider vinegar in a glass of water. The tea was without any sugar, sweeteners, milk or cream.

For activities, I only walked for one hour every day. I recommend you do Plank exercise for few minutes every day, but that I didn't do during my 3-month diet, I only started doing it recently after I finished the 3 months period.

As time went on, I started to feel less hungry, more energetic, slimmer, leaner and fitter. My dependency on food decreased significantly and my lust for the pleasure that food created diminished hugely.

By the end of the second month I started doing two meals a day. I ate the same amount of food with the same ingredients. I just shortened the eating window. It was at first 8 hours, then I decreased it to 6 hours, and I consumed my breakfast at 3 pm. Then I decreased it to 4 hours, and I consumed my first food of the day at 5 pm. I still ate salad, protein, eggs, nuts, and fruits. Now I eat on 2 hours window and fast for 22 hours every day, as I start eating 6:30 pm and stop eating 8:30 pm and sleep 9:30 pm. I never feel hungry unless I eat carbs.

I had digital scale and was weighting myself every day. I did the measuring every morning after I wake up, naked and done with bathroom activities, and before I drank anything. The first couple of weeks there was no change in my weight at all. Then the change started to take place.

My weight started to get down by one ounce daily for couple of weeks, then by two ounces, then by three, then by four, until the last month when I was losing weight by eight ounces on daily basis. Considering that I was consuming the same amount of food but in shorter and shorter period of time.

I consumed junk food few times on those 3 months, and when I consumed it, I gained weight not lost it. I ate pizza on one occasion, two times burger, I ate on one occasion fried chicken nuggets, and couple of times other fast food meals. I rarely ate bread or anything that had wheat in it. I ate rice on two occasions during that period.

I stopped adding sugar at all to any of my food and drinks. I didn't eat anything that had sugar in it. I was careful and cautious to know the components and ingredients of everything I buy. I stopped eating canned food, the exception was tuna only. I stopped eating or drinking any manufactured food. I only ate natural fresh foods.

Summarizing my plan will be as follow:

- ✓ I ate salad, eggs, protein, fruit, nuts, and other healthy fresh foods.
- ✓ I was on low-carb and high-fat diet.
- ✓ I stayed away from sugar, carbs, any food that included those.

- ✓ I Fasted for 16 hours and more, ate in 8 hours or less.
- ✓ I stopped all manufactured or canned foods, and rarely consumed junk or fast food.
- ✓ I walked for one hour a day.
- ✓ I prepared most of the meal days in advance and sticked to them and didn't eat more.
- ✓ I included organic super foods in my diet.
- ✓ I included natural organic fats with the protein.
- ✓ I used the air fryer to cook my protein.
- ✓ I drank water, coffee, tea, herbs; black without sugar, milk or cream.
- ✓ I used apple cider vinegar as an essential in my diet.
- ✓ I monitored my progress and didn't get disappointed when there were setbacks.

I recommend you take other vitamins supplement that will help you greatly in avoiding any side effects of the diet and improve your progress and help you achieve better results; however I didn't use any. Also exercise is important and staying active can be a factor in quicker results, but I didn't do that either.

The biggest problem you definitely will face is giving up on sugar, as it is proven to be an addictive substance. That is why it is added to almost every fast food meal and canned food and manufactured food ever created. It is a commercial cash cow that everyone is using to get people to buy and keep coming back. You must stop consuming it as it the number one factor in getting you fatter and less healthy.

Losing weight is psychological battle that you must end up on top of it. Commitment and disciplines are your best allies. You set your goal and make all possible sacrifices to achieve it. What I did was that I planned and determined what I would eat and when I would eat it before I started the day, and just followed the plan.

Benefits of my plan

Fasting is an ancient method humankind used since the dawn of history to survive dark times. It is a way of life in many religions. Our ancestors adapted it as a main approach to live a better life.

The human body by default is a surviving machine. It can withstand and adapt to extreme environment and unnormal life conditions. Fasting teach our bodies the most important lesson we are trying to convey here, which is food is not as important as what we make it to be.

Fasting trigger the body to be less dependent on outside sources of fuel and start using its reserves. Once the body recognizes that fasting has started and there is no food consumption upcoming, it will reprogram itself to start burning fats stored in the cells to supply itself with the energy it needs to survive the lack of food.

Engaging in intermittent fasting for long periods of time will make the body less and less dependent on food consumption. It will circulate and organize the fat burning mechanism for efficient reserving of energy the body needs to function properly. Fasting is our defense system against food enslavement and our attacking system against weight gain, diseases and other negative health issues.

That is why fasting is the best approach to weight loss. If done right, it will have a huge impact on your overall health in the best way possible.

Keto diet pushes the body to switch its source of energy from glucose as an energy source to the more efficient source of energy which is ketones. Our bodies love to run on ketones a lot more than glucose. Low carb high fat diets stimulate more ketones and less glucose in the body. Also that diet provide the body with so much important nutrition that are needed for better overall health.

Simply put, committing to combine the two together for a period of time will make your body go into beast mode.

Current global outbreak

There is no denial that this outbreak is getting spread faster and faster worldwide by the hour, and already was considered a pandemic. The good news is you can prevent infection, and if it happens you can recover. This is due to your health and how strong you are.

Keto and fasting help you greatly in achieving a healthy status that help you fight such diseases and infections. Both stimulate autophagy, make the body produce more of the growth hormone, and strengthen your immune system in a significant way. This is proven medically and scientifically.

The growth hormone is the compound in your body responsible for making you physically and mentally stronger. It enhances your overall health and help you get more powerful. This is crucial in combating all sorts of infections and illnesses.

Autophagy is a mechanism that helps you get rid of all your bad cells and unusable proteins and hormones. It acts as a cleansing tool the body uses to make itself function in an optimal way. Keto and fasting have a huge effect on initiating and strengthening autophagy. This is definitely an efficient way in protecting yourself from getting sick or infected and combating the symptoms and getting healed and recovered if you ever get infected.

The immune system is your number one protector, soldier and the shield that defends you in your battle against the current global outbreak and other diseases and infections. It is proven that fasting and keto will help you make your immune system functions in the best way possible. Fasting make your body goes into a defensive survival mode which makes your body produces more stronger white blood cells like crazy. Keto provide the white cells with all the nutrition, minerals and vitamins they need to function better. Those cells are the main component to combat and eradicate anything harmful to your body, especially outbreaks.

However, the development on the outbreak status is getting worse by the hour, and we must do what the experts are recommending. We should follow safety procedures and hygiene instructions like washing our hands, not touching anyone, keeping all surfaces around us clean, wearing masks, and other ways to prevent getting infected.

In those times in history, the strong survives and the weak perishes. We want everyone to be strong and survive, but some people are destined to be weak. To be stronger is to get in shape and eat healthy food and do exercise and commit to fasting. This way you are preparing yourself for survival.

If you start to have a healthy lifestyle and stick to it, your will shall manifest in the universe, and it will consider you as a stronger being who it can't mess with.

People over-react to this situation and consider only how many cases have died from the outbreak. For me, I look at the bright side and consider how many cases have recovered from it. Those recovered for sure had a better immune system and healthier overall body. Hope for the best but prepare for the worst.

My results

First thing that changed drastically for me was the hunger. Now I can go more than a day without eating anything, only I can survive the day on some tea and coffee and plenty of water. Hunger and cravings are now not an issue at all. I can go full day without eating at all as I did 24 hours fasting two times after I finished the 3 months plan. The hunger is no longer exists. This is due to the reduced amount of carbs and increased amount of fats I consume. Protein and fresh green veggies terminate the feeling of hunger, but sugars and carbs increase it.

That diet and fasting reprogrammed my mentality on how I perceived food and eating. Now I don't look to food as a pleasure, a joy, or a source of satisfaction, and not even as a source of fuel. I see it now as a medicine. I take food in to heal my body to make me stronger and healthier.

During that 3 months period I never got dizzy or fainted. Sometimes I felt cold hands and feet but that went off after few minutes. I never got sick since I started the program. I feel now invincible and bullet-proof.

My digestive system is working properly again. I have no problems at all in my stomach or guts. I don't feel pain anywhere in my body. I don't get bloating, inflammation or headaches anymore. I made blood, urine, stool, and x-ray tests after the three-month period, and the tests results showed increased improvements in my data. I have no more gout, high blood pressure, high cholesterol, or any digestive issue.

All my health problem related to consumption of food and drinks are fixed, except my non-alcoholic fatty liver disease. My liver has significant decreased amount of fat, but a fatty liver disease takes long time to be cured entirely. However I'm 100% sure that I'm on the right track to achieve that goal.

My energy is boosted hugely, I don't get tired that easy, and rarely gets exhausted. I'm lazy no more and that is helping me a lot in achieving many of my goals. I do more exercise now and I'm socially active more than ever. Fatigue is significantly reduced, and I rarely experience it.

Food no longer seduce me, and I can live without any temptations created by delicious fancy food. I can see any tasty, pretty looking dishes and meal, and smell that luring smell of restaurants and fast foods and never get the urge to eat them or even come close. I was slave to food consumption, now I'm free of it. Food controlled my life for so long, and now I control it.

By the end of second month, I started to sleep earlier, and by the end of the third month I was sleeping at 9:30 pm and wake up 5 am. Before the diet, it was very hard for me to sleep and wake up early. But by the end of the third I was able to sleep and wake up on command. I didn't have any trouble sleeping, I just put my head on the pillow and sleep like a little baby. I set my alarm and wake up anytime I want fresh and active without any tiredness.

word of advice to you as I'm your fellow human been.

I'm not here to sell you other things. This eBook is not a gateway to other offers, products, services, or other eBooks I sell that I want you to buy. You will not find here a link to another offer that has a link to another offer that has a link to another offer. I'm not another guru who tries to use you and benefit from you. I'm not a personal trainer, nutritionist, or health specialist.

I'm here to tell you my story, my experience, and my case study. I'm here to open my heart and give you all the information I have on the subject in all honesty and completely.

People in this world are suffering from what they put in their mouths. I think 95% of world diseases are results of food and drinks. The corporate machine wants us to eat all the time, then get sick, then use their medical system and buy their medicine. Where you can naturally cure yourself by eating and drinking the right healthy food. Natural foods are proven to prevent and heal most of our illness.

I highly recommend you subscribe to the before-mentioned YouTube channels for more clarifications on all the aspect of my plan. You will find so much more information online where you can find legitimate sources of information. I can't stress enough how you should not take my words literally, but to go out there and find your own path.

Our bodies are a miracle that was created to achieve excellence and we degraded and disrespected it by eating and drinking garbage, only because it tastes good and satisfy our need. Food can be considered by some as one of life pleasures, and sure it is. However it can be considered this way and be healthy and benefit us at the same time. We have in our body a "survival mode" that gets activated when fasting, and that mode help our body greatly in staying in shape and combating diseases.

I urge you to eat healthy food, fresh fruits and vegetables. Drink tea and herbs. Eat eggs, boiled, grilled or steamed protein, like fish, beef and chicken. Eat a lot of avocado, broccoli, nuts, cruciferous vegetables. Use olive and coconuts oils, and organic butter, and also use apple cider vinegar on daily basis.

Your body and your health are your most valuable asset. Treat it right, respect it, cherish it. Life will be a lot better if you take good care of your body. Control the fuel you give to your body. Manage what you put in your mouth. Living unhealthy lifestyle will make you miserable, get you to waste your money on unnecessary food and drinks and medicine.

In your war against food control and in your struggle against weight loss, sugar is your number one enemy. You must fight it with all you have, and you must win. It is the main cause of cravings and hunger, and number one factor in weight gain.

Life is short as they say, and the best way to enjoy it is to be happy. One of the ways to be happy is that you need to be satisfied with yourself. To achieve satisfaction is to look in the mirror and say "wow... I really have a fit and healthy body".